Everything You Need to Know About Ankylosing Spondylitis

Ankylosing spondylitis is a type of arthritis that causes inflammation in the joints and ligaments of the spine. Normally, the joints and ligaments in the spine help us move and bend. If you have ankylosing spondylitis, over time, the inflammation in the joints and tissues of the spine can cause stiffness. In severe cases, this may cause the vertebrae (bones in the spine) to fuse (grow together). When the vertebrae fuse, it can lead to a rigid and inflexible spine.

Many people with ankylosing spondylitis have mild episodes of back pain and stiffness that come and go. But others have severe, ongoing pain with loss of flexibility in the spine. In addition, other symptoms may develop if other areas of the body— such as the hips, ribs, shoulders, knees, ankles, and feet—are affected by the disease.

There is no cure for ankylosing spondylitis. Doctors recommend treatments that may include exercise and medications to help manage pain, control inflammation, improve posture and body position, and slow the progression of the disease. With treatment, most people with ankylosing spondylitis can have productive lives.

Who Gets Ankylosing Spondylitis?

Anyone can get ankylosing spondylitis; however, certain factors may increase your risk for developing the disease. These factors include:

- **Family history and genetics.** If you have a family history of ankylosing spondylitis, you are more likely to develop the disease.
- **Age.** Most people develop symptoms of ankylosing spondylitis before age 45. However, some people develop the disease when they are children or teens.
- **Sex.** Men are more likely to have ankylosing spondylitis than women.
- **Other conditions.** People who have Crohn's disease, ulcerative colitis, or psoriasis may be more likely to develop the disease.

Symptoms of Ankylosing Spondylitis

The most common symptom of ankylosing spondylitis is lower back and/or hip pain and stiffness. Over time, the symptoms may progress to other areas of the spine. The pain typically worsens during periods of rest or inactivity, which may cause some people to experience more pain during the middle of the night or after prolonged sitting.

Everything You Need to Know About Ankylosing Spondylitis

Causes ◆ Symptoms ◆ Treatment

Watch a video version:
https://www.youtube.com/watch?v=enHpxaj2glg

This book is based on information and recommendations by the Department of Health, United States government.

Created By The Bizmove Health Team

Disclaimer

All the content found in this book was created for informational purposes only. The Content is not intended to be a substitute for professional medical advice, diagnosis, or treatment. Always seek the advice of your physician or other qualified health provider with any questions you may have regarding a medical condition. Never disregard professional medical advice or delay in seeking it because of something you have read in this book.

ISBN: 9798746871565

Usually, moving and exercise can help improve pain.

Symptoms of ankylosing spondylitis vary from person to person. Some people have mild episodes of pain that come and go, while others will have chronic, severe pain. The symptoms of ankylosing spondylitis, whether mild or severe, may worsen in "flares" and improve during periods of remission.

Because the disease can affect other areas of the body, other symptoms may develop and may include:

- Pain, stiffness, and inflammation in other joints, such as the ribs, shoulders, knees, or feet.
- Difficulty taking deep breaths if the joints connecting the ribs are affected.
- Vision changes and eye pain due to uveitis, which is inflammation of the eye.
- Fatigue, or feeling very tired.
- Loss of appetite and weight loss.
- Skin rashes.
- Abdominal pain and loose bowel movements.

Causes of Ankylosing Spondylitis

Researchers do not know the cause of ankylosing spondylitis. However, studies show that both genes and environment may lead to the development of the disease. Researchers know that the HLA-B27 gene increases the risk of developing ankylosing spondylitis, but this does not mean you will get the disease if you have the gene. Many people have the gene and never develop ankylosing spondylitis, which tells researchers that environmental factors also play a role.

Researchers continue to discover many other gene variations that may cause the disease; however, HLA-B27 is the primary gene that increases your risk for developing ankylosing spondylitis.

Diagnosis of Ankylosing Spondylitis

To diagnose ankylosing spondylitis, your doctor will ask you about your medical history and perform a physical exam. Your doctor may order imaging studies and lab tests to help confirm a diagnosis.

Medical and Family History

Your doctor may ask about your medical and family history, including questions such as:

- How long have you had pain?
- Where is your pain?
- What makes the pain better or worse?
- Does anyone in your family have a history of back pain, joint pain, or arthritis?

Physical Exam

A physical exam may include:

- Examining your joints, including your spine, pelvis, heels, and chest.
- Watching how you move and bend in different directions, checking for flexibility.
- Asking you to breathe deeply to check for rib stiffness and inflammation.

Imaging Studies

Your doctor may order imaging studies to help diagnose ankylosing spondylitis:

- X-rays help doctors see joint changes. However, you may have the disease for years before the changes show on x-rays. Doctors may use x-rays to monitor the progression of the disease or to rule out other causes for the joint pain.
- Magnetic resonance imaging (MRI) uses energy from a powerful magnet to produce signals that create a series of cross-sectional images. These images or "slices" are analyzed by a computer to produce an image of the joint. MRI can help diagnose ankylosing spondylitis in the early stages of the disease.

Your doctor may use both x-rays and MRIs to follow the progression of your disease.

Lab tests

At this time, no single test diagnoses ankylosing spondylitis. Your doctor may order a blood test to check for the HLA-B27 gene, which is present in most people with the disease. You may have the HLA-B27 gene and never develop ankylosing spondylitis, but it can give doctors more information when making a diagnosis.

Treatment of Ankylosing Spondylitis

There is no cure for ankylosing spondylitis; however, your doctor will work with you to help manage the disease. The goals of treatment include:

- Relieve symptoms.
- Help maintain proper posture.
- Slow the progression of the disease.

In most cases, treatment includes medication and physical therapy. Sometimes, people with severe disease need surgery to repair joint damage.

Medications

Most people with ankylosing spondylitis take medications, which may include one or more of the following:

- Over-the-counter anti-inflammatory medications to relieve pain and inflammation are commonly used to treat ankylosing spondylitis.
- Biologic medications target specific immune messages and interrupt the signal, helping to decrease or stop inflammation. These medications may be prescribed if your disease is unresponsive to other treatments.
- Corticosteroids can help decrease inflammation and provide some pain relief. They are usually injected into the joint. Because they are potent drugs, your doctor will determine how much and how many injections you should receive to achieve the desired benefit.

Physical Therapy

Your doctor may recommend physical therapy to help:

- Relieve pain.
- Strengthen back and neck muscles.

- Improve core and abdominal muscle strength because these muscles provide support for your back.
- Improve posture.
- Maintain and improve flexibility in joints.

A physical therapist can recommend the best sleeping positions and an exercise program. Because your symptoms may worsen when inactive or at rest, it's important to stay active and exercise regularly.

Surgery

If you have severe joint damage and you are unable to participate in your daily activities, your doctor may recommend surgery. Surgery is not for everyone. You and your doctor can discuss the options and choose what is right for you.

Your doctor will consider the following before recommending surgery:

- Your overall health.
- The condition of the affected bone or joint.
- The risks and benefits of the surgery.

Types of surgery may include joint repairs and joint replacements.

Rarely, some people may have surgery to correct or straighten the spine or repair fractures (breaks) in the vertebrae.

Who Treats Ankylosing Spondylitis?

Diagnosing and treating ankylosing spondylitis may require a team of health care professionals. These may include:

- Rheumatologists, who specialize in arthritis and other diseases of the bones, joints, and muscles.
- Dermatologists, who specialize in conditions of the skin, hair, and nails.
- Gastroenterologists, who specialize in conditions of the digestive system.
- Mental health professionals, who help people cope with difficulties in the home and workplace that may result from their medical conditions.
- Nurse educators, who specialize in helping people understand their overall condition and set up their treatment plans.
- Occupational therapists, who teach ways to protect joints, minimize pain, perform activities of daily living, and conserve energy.
- Ophthalmologists, who specialize in conditions of the eye.
- Orthopaedic surgeons, who specialize in treatment and surgery for bone and joint diseases.

- Physiatrists (physical, medicine, and rehabilitation specialists), who supervise exercise programs.
- Physical therapists, who help improve joint function.
- Primary care doctors, such as a family physician or internal medicine specialist, who coordinates care between the different health providers and treats other problems as they arise.
- Psychologists or social workers, who help with psychosocial challenges caused by medical conditions.

Living With Ankylosing Spondylitis

Research shows that people who take part in their own care report less pain and make fewer doctor visits. They also enjoy a better quality of life.

Self-care can help you play a role in managing your ankylosing spondylitis and improving your health. You can:

- Learn about the disease and its treatments.
- Communicate well with your health care team so you can have more control over your disease.
- Reach out for support to help cope with the physical, emotional, and mental effects of ankylosing spondylitis.

Participating in your care can help build confidence

in your ability to perform day-to-day activities, allowing you to lead a full, active, and independent life.

The following lifestyle changes and activities can help improve your ability to function on your own and maintain a positive outlook.

- **Exercise.** Exercise is important for maintaining healthy and strong muscles, preserving joint mobility, and maintaining flexibility. In addition to an exercise program, your doctor may recommend low-impact exercises, such as water exercise programs. Talk to your health care providers before beginning any exercise program. Exercise can help:
  - Improve your sleep.
  - Decrease pain.
  - Keep a positive attitude.
  - Maintain a healthy weight.
- **Posture.** Another important thing you can do for yourself is to practice good posture. Your physical therapist and doctors can give you tips and exercises to help maintain and improve your posture. Practicing good posture can help you avoid some of the complications that can occur with ankylosing spondylitis.
- **Support or assistive devices.** Using a cane or walker can help you move around safely, provide stability, and lower pain. If you have trouble

bending due to spine stiffness, try using a device to grab or pick up items.

- **Monitoring of symptoms.** It is important to monitor your symptoms for any changes or the development of new symptoms. Understanding your symptoms and how they may change can help you and your doctor manage your pain when you have a flare.
- **Stress management.** The emotions you may feel because of your disease, along with any pain, physical limitations, and the unpredictable nature of flares, can increase your stress level. Although there is no evidence that stress plays a role in your disease, it can make living with ankylosing spondylitis more difficult. Ways to cope with stress can include:
    - Use relaxation techniques such as deep breathing, meditating, or listening to quiet sounds or music.
    - Try movement exercise programs, such as yoga and tai chi.
- **Mental health management.** If you feel alone, anxious, or depressed about having ankylosing spondylitis, talk to your doctor or mental health professional. Keep the lines of communication open. Talk to family and friends about your disease. You may find it helpful to join an online or community support group.

- **Healthy diet.** A healthy diet is good for everyone, and it may be very helpful if you have ankylosing spondylitis. There is no specific diet for people with ankylosing spondylitis, but keeping a healthy weight is important. It reduces stress on painful joints.
- **Smoking.** If you smoke, quit. Ankylosing spondylitis is more severe in people who smoke, and smoking blunts the effect of treatment. In addition, if you have ankylosing spondylitis in the chest or ribs, smoking can compromise your lung function even more. Smoking is also a risk factor for progression of disease.

Appendix A: Guide to Better Living

Note: Always consult your physician before making any changes to your diet, physical activity or life style.

Is your health condition requires that you make changes to your diet, physical activity, or life style? Are you thinking about being more active? Have you been trying to cut back on less healthy foods? Are you starting to eat better and move more but having a hard time sticking with these changes?

Old habits die hard. Changing your habits is a process that involves several stages. Sometimes it takes a while before changes become new habits. And, you may face roadblocks along the way.

Adopting new, healthier habits may protect you from serious health problems. New habits, like healthy eating and regular physical activity, may also help you manage your weight and have more energy. After a while, if you stick with these changes, they may become part of your daily routine.

The information below outlines four stages you may go through when changing your health habits or behavior. You will also find tips to help you improve your eating, physical activity habits, and overall health. The four stages of changing a health behavior are

- contemplation
- preparation
- action
- maintenance

What stage of change are you in?

Contemplation: "I'm thinking about it."

In this first stage, you are thinking about change and becoming motivated to get started.

You might be in this stage if you

- have been considering change but are not quite ready to start
- believe that your health, energy level, or overall well-being will improve if you develop new habits
- are not sure how you will overcome the roadblocks that may keep you from starting to change

Preparation: "I have made up my mind to take action."

In this next stage, you are making plans and thinking of specific ideas that will work for you.

You might be in this stage if you

- have decided that you are going to change and are ready to take action
- have set some specific goals that you would like to meet
- are getting ready to put your plan into action

Action: "I have started to make changes."

In this third stage, you are acting on your plan and making the changes you set out to achieve.

You might be in this stage if you

- have been making eating, physical activity, and other behavior changes in the last 6 months or so
- are adjusting to how it feels to eat healthier, be more active, and make other changes such as getting more sleep or reducing screen time
- have been trying to overcome things that sometimes block your success

Maintenance: "I have a new routine."

In this final stage, you have become used to your changes and have kept them up for more than 6 months.

You might be in this stage if

- your changes have become a normal part of your routine
- you have found creative ways to stick with your routine
- you have had slip-ups and setbacks but have been able to get past them and make progress

Did you find your stage of change? Read on for ideas about what you can do next.

Contemplation: Are you thinking of making changes?

Making the leap from thinking about change to taking action can be hard and may take time. Asking yourself about the pros (benefits) and cons (things that get in the way) of changing your habits may be helpful. How would life be better if you made some changes?

Think about how the benefits of healthy eating or regular physical activity might relate to your overall health. For example, suppose your blood glucose, also called blood sugar, is a bit high and you have a parent, brother, or sister who has type 2 diabetes. This means you also may develop type 2 diabetes. You may find that it is easier to be physically active and eat healthy knowing that it may help control blood glucose and protect you from a serious disease.

You may learn more about the benefits of changing your eating and physical activity habits from a health care professional. This knowledge may help you take action.

Look at the lists of pros and cons below. Find the items you believe are true for you. Think about factors that are important to you.

Healthy Eating

Pros

- have more energy
- improve my health
- lower my risk for health problems
- maintain a healthy weight
- feel proud of myself
- set an example for friends and family

Cons

- may spend more money and time on food
- may need to cook more often at home
- may need to eat less of foods I love
- may need to buy different foods
- may need to convince my family that we all have to eat healthier foods

Physical Activity

Pros

- improve my health
- reduce my risk for serious health problems
- feel better about myself
- become stronger
- have fun
- take time to care for myself
- meet new people and spend time with them
- have more energy
- maintain a healthy weight
- become a role model for others

Cons

- takes too much time and energy
- it is too hot or cold outside
- feel self-conscious
- am nervous about my health
- could hurt myself
- am not good at being active
- do not know what to do
- have no one to be active with
- am not young or fit enough
- keeps me from family and friends

Preparation: Have you made up your mind?

If you are in the preparation stage, you are about to take action. To get started, look at your list of pros and cons. How can you make a plan and act on it?

The chart below lists common roadblocks you may face and possible solutions to overcome roadblocks as you begin to change your habits. Think about these things as you make your plan.

Roadblock: I don't have time.

Solution: Make your new healthy habit a priority. Fit in physical activity whenever and wherever you can. Try taking the stairs or getting off the bus a stop early if it is safe to do so. Set aside one grocery shopping day a week, and make healthy meals that you can freeze and eat later when you don't have time to cook.

Roadblock: Healthy habits cost too much.

Solution: You can walk around the mall, a school track, or a local park for free. Eat healthy on a budget by buying in bulk and when items are on sale, and by choosing frozen or canned fruits and vegetables.

Roadblock: I can't make this change alone.

Solution: Recruit others to be active with you, which will help you stay motivated and safe. Consider signing up for a fun fitness class like salsa dancing. Get your family or coworkers on the healthy eating bandwagon. Plan healthy meals together with your family, or start a healthy potluck once a week at work.

Roadblock: I don't like physical activity.

Solution: Forget the old notion that being physically active means lifting weights in a gym. You can be active in many ways, including dancing, walking, or gardening. Make your own list of options that appeal to you. Explore options you never thought about, and stick with what you enjoy.

Roadblock: I don't like healthy foods.

Solution: Try making your old favorite recipes in healthier new ways. For example, you can trim fat from meats and reduce the amount of butter, sugar, and salt you cook with. Use low-fat cheeses or milk rather than whole-milk foods. Add a cup or two of broccoli, carrots, or spinach to casseroles or pasta.

Once you have made up your mind to change your habits, make a plan and set goals for taking action. Here are some ideas for making your plan:

- learn more about healthy eating (https://www.myplate.gov/)
- learn more about being active (see appendix B)
- make lists of
    - healthy foods that you like or may need to eat more of—or more often
    - foods you love that you may need to eat less often
    - things you could do to be more physically active
    - fun activities you like and could do more often, such as dancing

After making your plan, start setting goals for putting your plan into action. Start with small changes. For example, "I'm going to walk for 10 minutes, three times a week." What is the one step you can take right away?

Action: Have you started to make changes?

You are making real changes to your lifestyle, which is fantastic! To stick with your new habits

- review your plan
- look at the goals you set and how well you are meeting them
- overcome roadblocks by planning ahead for setbacks
- reward yourself for your hard work

Track your progress

- Tracking your progress helps you spot your strengths, find areas where you can improve, and stay on course. Record not only what you did, but how you felt while doing it—your feelings can play a role in making your new habits stick.
- Recording your progress may help you stay focused and catch setbacks in meeting your goals. Remember that a setback does not mean you have failed. All of us experience setbacks. The key is to get back on track as soon as you can.
- You can track your progress with online tools such as the NIH Body Weight Planner (https://www.youtube.com/watch?v=v1gluQwieog). The NIH Body Weight Planner lets you tailor your calorie and physical activity plans to reach your personal goals within a specific time period.

Overcome roadblocks

- Remind yourself why you want to be healthier. Perhaps you want the energy to play with your nieces and nephews or to be able to carry your own grocery bags. Recall your reasons for making changes when slip-ups occur. Decide to take the first step to get back on track.

- Problem-solve to "outsmart" roadblocks. For example, plan to walk indoors, such as at a mall, on days when bad weather keeps you from walking outside.
- Ask a friend or family member for help when you need it, and always try to plan ahead. For example, if you know that you will not have time to be physically active after work, go walking with a coworker at lunch or start your day with an exercise video.

Reward yourself

- After reaching a goal or milestone, allow for a nonfood reward such as new workout gear or a new workout device. Also consider posting a message on social media to share your success with friends and family.
- Choose rewards carefully. Although you should be proud of your progress, keep in mind that a high-calorie treat or a day off from your activity routine are not the best rewards to keep you healthy.
- Pat yourself on the back. When negative thoughts creep in, remind yourself how much good you are doing for your health by moving more and eating healthier.

Maintenance: Have you created a new routine?

Make your future a healthy one. Remember that eating healthy, getting regular physical activity, and other healthy habits are lifelong behaviors, not one-time events. Always keep an eye on your efforts and seek ways to deal with the planned and unplanned changes in life.

Now that healthy eating and regular physical activity are part of your routine, keep things interesting, avoid slip-ups, and find ways to cope with what life throws at you.

Add variety and stay motivated

Mix up your routine with new physical activities and goals, physical activity buddies, foods, recipes, and rewards.

Deal with unexpected setbacks

Plan ahead to avoid setbacks. For example, find other ways to be active in case of bad weather, injury, or other issues that arise. Think of ways to eat healthy when traveling or dining out, like packing healthy snacks while on the road or sharing an entrée with a friend in a restaurant.

If you do have a setback, don't give up. Setbacks happen to everyone. Regroup and focus on meeting your goals again as soon as you can.

Challenge yourself!

Revisit your goals and think of ways to expand them. For example, if you are comfortable walking 5 days a week, consider adding strength training twice a week. If you have limited your saturated fat intake by eating less fried foods, try cutting back on added sugars, too. Small changes can lead to healthy habits worth keeping.

**When The Going Gets Tough,
Put One Foot in Front of The
Other and Just Keep Going.
Don't Give Up!**

Appendix B: How to Stay Active

Note: Always consult your physician before making any changes to your diet, physical activity or life style.

Physical activity may seem hard if you're overweight. You may get short of breath or tired quickly. Finding or affording the right clothes and equipment may be frustrating. Or, perhaps you may not feel comfortable working out in front of others.

The good news is you can overcome these challenges. Not only can you be active at any size, you can have fun and feel good at the same time.

Can anyone be active?

Research strongly shows that physical activity is safe for almost everyone. The health benefits of physical activity far outweigh the risks.

The activities discussed here are safe for most people. If you have problems moving or staying steady on your feet, or if you get out of breath easily, talk with a health care professional before you start. You also should talk with a health care professional if you are unsure of your health, have any concerns that physical activity may be unsafe for you, or have

- a chronic disease such as diabetes, high blood pressure, or heart disease
- a bone or joint problem—for example, in your back, knee, or hip—that could get worse if you change your physical activity level

Why should I be active?

Being active may help you live longer and protect you from developing serious health problems, such as type 2 diabetes, heart disease, stroke, and certain types of cancer. Regular physical activity is linked to many health benefits, such as

- lower blood pressure and blood glucose, or blood sugar
- healthy bones, muscles, and joints
- a strong heart and lungs
- better sleep at night and improved mood

The Physical Activity Guidelines for Americans define regular physical activity as at least 150 minutes a week of moderate-intensity aerobic activity, such as brisk walking. Brisk walking is a pace of 3 miles per hour or faster. A moderate-intensity activity makes you breathe harder but does not overwork or overheat you. You should also do muscle-strengthening activities at least 2 days a week.

You may reach this goal by starting with 5 minutes

of physical activity several times a day, 5 to 6 days a week. You could then gradually work up to 10 minutes per session, 3 times a day. If you do even more activity, you may gain even more health benefits.

When combined with healthy eating, regular physical activity may also help you control your weight. However, research shows that even if you can't lose weight or maintain your weight loss, you still can enjoy important health benefits from regular physical activity.

Physical activity also can be a lot of fun if you do activities you enjoy and are active with other people. Being active with others may give you a chance to meet new people or spend more time with family and friends. You also may inspire and motivate one another to get and stay active.

What do I need to know about becoming active?

Choosing physical activities that match your fitness level and health goals can help you stay motivated and keep you from getting hurt. You may feel some minor discomfort or muscle soreness when you first become active. These feelings should go away as you get used to your activity. However, if you feel sick to your stomach or have pain, you may have done too much. Go easier and then slowly build up your activity level. Some activities, such as walking or swimming, are less likely to cause injuries.

If you have been inactive, start slowly and see how you feel. Gradually increase how long and how often you are active. If you need guidance, check with a health care or certified fitness professional.

Here are some tips for staying safe during physical activity:

- Wear the proper safety gear, such as a bike helmet if you are bicycling.
- Make sure any sports equipment you use works and fits properly.
- Look for safe places to be active. For instance, walk in well-lit areas where other people are around. Be active with a friend or group.
- Stay hydrated to replace the body fluids you lose through sweating and to prevent you from getting overheated.
- If you are active outdoors, protect yourself from the sun with sunscreen and a hat or protective visor and clothing.
- Wear enough clothing to keep warm in cold or windy weather. Layers are best.

If you don't feel right, stop your activity. If you have any of the following warning signs, stop and seek help right away:

- pain, tightness, or pressure in your chest or neck, shoulder, or arm
- extreme shortness of breath
- dizziness or sickness

Check with a health care professional about what to do if you have any of these warning signs. If your activity is causing pain in your joints, feet, ankles, or legs, you also should consult a health care professional to see if you may need to change the type or amount of activity you are doing.

What kinds of activities can I do?

You don't need to be an athlete or have special skills or equipment to make physical activity part of your life. Many types of activities you do every day, such as walking your dog or going up and down steps at home or at work, may help improve your health.

Try different activities you enjoy. If you like an activity, you're more likely to stick with it. Anything that gets you moving around, even for a few minutes at a time, is a healthy start to getting fit.

Walking

Walking is free and easy to do—and you can do it

almost anywhere. Walking will help you

- burn calories
- improve your fitness
- lift your mood
- strengthen your bones and muscles

If you are concerned about safety, try walking in a shopping mall or park where it is well lit and other people are around. Many malls and parks have benches where you can take a quick break. Walking with a friend or family member is safer than walking alone and may provide the social support you need to meet your activity goals.

If you don't have time for a long walk, take several short walks instead. For example, instead of a 30-minute walk, add three 10-minute walks to your day. Shorter spurts of activity are easier to fit into a busy schedule.

Walking tips

- Wear comfortable, well-fitting walking shoes with a lot of support, and socks that absorb sweat.
- Dress for the weather if you are walking outdoors. In cold weather, wear layers of clothing you can remove if you start getting too warm. In hot weather, protect yourself against the sun and heat.

- Warm up by walking more slowly for the first few minutes. Cool down by slowing your pace.

Dancing

Dancing can be a lot of fun while it tones your muscles, strengthens your heart and lungs, and boosts your mood. You can dance at a health club, dance studio, or even at home. Just turn on some lively music and start moving. You also can dance to a video on your TV or computer.

If you have trouble standing on your feet for a long time, try dancing while sitting down. Chair dancing lets you move your arms and legs to music while taking the weight off your feet.

Bicycling

Riding a bicycle spreads your weight among your arms, back, and hips. For outdoor biking, you may want to try a mountain bike. Mountain bikes have wider tires and are sturdier than bikes with thinner tires. You can buy a larger seat to make biking more comfortable.

For indoor biking, you may want to try a recumbent bike. On this type of bike, you sit lower to the ground with your legs reaching forward to the pedals. Your body is in more of a reclining position, which may feel better than sitting straight up. The seat on a recumbent bike is also wider than the seat on a regular bike.

If you decide to buy a bike, check how much weight it can support to make sure it is safe for you.

Workout clothing tips

- Clothes made of fabrics that absorb sweat are best for working out.
- Comfortable, lightweight clothes allow you to move more easily.
- Tights or spandex shorts are the best bottoms to wear to prevent inner-thigh chafing.
- Women should wear a bra that provides extra support during physical activity.

Water workouts

Swimming and water workouts put less stress on your joints than walking, dancing, or biking. If your feet, back, or joints hurt when you stand, water activities may be best for you. If you feel self-conscious about wearing a bathing suit, you can wear shorts and a T-shirt while you swim.

Exercising in water

- Lets you be more flexible. You can move your body in water in ways you may not be able to on land.

- Reduces your risk of hurting yourself. Water provides a natural cushion, which keeps you from pounding or jarring your joints.
- Helps prevent sore muscles.
- Keeps you cool, even when you are working hard.

You don't need to know how to swim to work out in water. You can do shallow- or deep-water exercises at either end of the pool without swimming. For instance, you can do laps while holding onto a kickboard and kicking your feet. You also can walk or jog across the width of the pool while moving your arms.

For shallow-water workouts, the water level should be between your waist and chest. During deep-water workouts, most of your body is underwater. For safety and comfort, wear a foam belt or life jacket.

Tips for protecting your hair

If you're worried that pool water will damage or mess up your hair, try these tips:

- Use a swim cap to help protect your hair from pool chemicals and getting wet.
- Wear a natural hairstyle, short braids, locs, or twists, which may be easier to style after a water workout.

- Buy a shampoo to remove chlorine buildup, available at most drug stores, if your hair feels dry or damaged after a pool workout.

Strength training

Strength training involves using free weights, weightlifting machines, resistance bands, or your own body weight to make your muscles stronger. Lower-body strength training will improve your balance and prevent falls.

Strength training may help you

- build and maintain strong muscles as you get older
- continue to perform activities of daily living, such as carrying groceries or moving furniture
- keep your bones strong, which may help prevent osteoporosis and fractures

If you are just starting out, using a weightlifting machine may be safer than dumbbells. As you get fit, you may want to add free-weight exercises with dumbbells.

You do not need a weight bench or large dumbbells to do strength training at home. You can use a pair of hand weights to do bicep curls. You can also use your own body weight: for example, get up and down from a chair.

Proper form is very important when lifting weights. You may hurt yourself if you don't lift weights properly. You may want to schedule a session with a certified fitness professional to learn which exercises to do and how to do them safely. Check with your health insurer about whether your health plan covers these services.

If you decide to buy a home gym, check how much weight it can support to make sure it is safe for you.

Strength-training tips

- Aim for at least 2 days per week of strengthen-training activities.
- Try to perform each exercise 8 to 12 times. If that's too hard, the weight you are lifting is too heavy. If it's too easy, your weight is too light.
- Try to exercise all the major muscle groups. These groups include the muscles of the legs, hips, chest, back, abdomen, shoulders, and arms.
- Don't work the same muscles 2 days in a row. Your muscles need time to recover.

Mind and body exercise

Your local hospital or fitness, recreation, or community center may offer classes such as yoga, tai chi, or Pilates. You also may find some of these workouts online and can download them to a computer, smart phone, or other device. These types of activities may help you

- become stronger and more flexible
- feel more relaxed
- improve balance and posture

Your local hospital or fitness, recreation, or community center may offer classes such as yoga, tai chi, or Pilates.

These classes also can be a lot of fun and add variety to your workout routine. If some movements are hard to do or you have injuries you are concerned about, talk with the instructor about how to adapt the exercises and poses to meet your needs—or start with a beginner's class.

Daily life activities

Daily life activities, such as cleaning out the attic or washing the car, are great ways to get moving. Small changes can add more physical activity to your day and improve your health. Try these:

- Take 2- to 3-minute walking breaks at work several times a day, if possible.
- Stand, walk, or stretch in place during TV commercials.
- Take the stairs instead of the elevator or escalator whenever you can.

- Park farther from where you are going and walk the rest of the way.

Even a shopping trip can be exercise because it provides a chance to walk and carry your bags. Chores such as mowing the lawn, raking leaves, and gardening also count.

Where can I be active?

You can find many fun places to be active. Having more than one place may keep you from getting bored. Here are some options:

- Join or take a class at a local fitness, recreation, or community center.
- Enjoy the outdoors by taking a hike or going for a walk in a safe local park, neighborhood, or mall.
- Work out in the comfort of your own home with a workout video or by finding a fitness channel on your TV, tablet, or other mobile device.

Tips for choosing a fitness center

- Make sure the center has exercise equipment for people who weigh more and staff to show you how to use it.
- Ask if the center has any special classes for people just starting out, older adults, or people with mobility or health issues.

- See if you can try out the center or take a class before you join.
- Try to find a center close to work or home. The quicker and easier the center is to get to, the better your chances of using it often.
- Make sure you understand the rules for joining and ending your membership, what your membership fee covers, any related costs, and the days and hours of operation.

How can I get past my roadblocks?

You most likely will face roadblocks that keep you from meeting your physical activity goals. Think about what keeps you from being active, then try to come up with creative ways to address those roadblocks. Here are a few examples to help you get started:

Barrier: I don't have enough time.

Solution: Instead of doing one long workout session, build in three 10-minute bursts of activity during your day, such as a brisk walk. Even standing up instead of sitting at your desk has benefits.

Barrier: I just don't like exercise.

Solution: Good news! You don't have to run a marathon or go to the gym all the time to benefit from being active. To make physical activity more fun, try something you enjoy doing, such as dancing to the radio or taking a yoga class with friends. Many people find they start to like exercise better the more they do it.

Barrier: I'm worried about my health or getting hurt.

Solution: If you have a hard time being active because of your health, talk with a health care professional first. A certified fitness professional can also guide you on how to be active safely.

Barrier: I feel self-conscious working out in front of others.

Solution: Start being active at home until you feel more confident. Be active with friends who will support and encourage you.

How can I stick with my physical activity plan?

Sticking with a plan to be physically active can be a challenge. Online tools such as the NIH Body Weight Planner (https://www.youtube.com/watch?v=v1gluQwieog) can help. The NIH Body Weight Planner lets you tailor your calorie and physical activity plans to reach your personal goals within a specific time period.

You also can download fitness apps that let you enter information to track your progress using a computer or smart phone or other mobile device.

Devices you can wear, such as pedometers and fitness trackers, may help you count steps, calories, and minutes of physical activity. Trackers can help you set goals and monitor progress. You wear most of these devices on your wrist like a watch, or clipped to your clothing.

Keeping an activity journal is another good way to help you stay motivated and on track to reach your fitness goals.

Set goals. As you track your activity, try to set specific short- and long-term goals. For example, instead of "I will be more active," set a goal such as "I will take a walk after lunch at least 2 days a week." Getting started with a doable goal is a good way to form a new habit. A short-term goal may be to walk 5 to 10 minutes, 5 days a week. A long-term goal may be to do at least 150 minutes of moderate-intensity physical activity a week.

Get support. Ask a family member or friend to be active with you. Your workout buddy can help make your activities more fun and can cheer you on and help you meet your goals.

Track progress. You may not feel as though you

are making progress, but when you look back at where you started, you may be pleasantly surprised. Making regular activity part of your life is a big step. Start slowly and praise yourself for every goal you set and achieve.

Review your goals. Did you meet your goals? If not, why? Are they doable? Did you hit a roadblock trying to meet your goal? What will you do differently next week? Brainstorm some options to overcome future roadblocks. Ask a friend or family member to help support your goals.

Pick nonfood rewards. Whether your goal is to be active 15 minutes a day, to walk farther than you did last week, or simply to stay positive, recognizing your efforts is an important part of staying on track. Decide how you will reward yourself. Some ideas for rewards include getting new music to charge you up or buying new workout gear.

Be patient with yourself. Don't get discouraged if you have setbacks from time to time. If you can't achieve your goal the first time or can only stick to your goals for part of the week, remind yourself that this is all part of establishing new habits.

Look ahead. Try to focus on what you will do differently moving forward, rather than on what went wrong. Pat yourself on the back for trying.

Most importantly, don't give up. Any movement, even for a short time, is a good thing. Each activity you add to your life is another step toward a healthier you.